Your Weight Loss & Keto Diet

Change Your Diet Plan with Intermittent Fasting through Ketogenic Diet Stay Healthy Make Your Diets at Home Fast

Lucia Palomar

Introduction

The demands of lifestyles today condition and determine to a certain extent all our habits. From how we sleep, how we organize, how we work and study. Our food also does not escape this rapid onslaught of modern times in which we are permanently over stimulated and hyperconnected. At a time when efficiency and effectiveness predominate in all aspects of our society, it is not surprising that methods were adopted that seek to fit in with the modern human being.

Intermittent fasting has catapulted in recent years into dietary trends as one of the most effective and useful methods to improve our health and performance in all areas of our life. The benefits to our health, whether we seek to lose weight or simply improve our well-being and happiness, are constantly reaffirmed by some experts and by people who prefer to adopt this new eating habit, especially if accompanied by the ketogenic diet to boost, improve and accelerate the outcomes of intermittent fasting.

With professional help, with the knowledge of how our body as a whole works, as an open and living system, and plans suited to one goal or another, the following text seeks to shed light on the characteristics of intermittent fasting as a lifestyle, benefits and disadvantages, important considerations and synergies between our physical and mental health, as important as interdependent to ensure the improvement of our well-being and improve our ability to be happy both physically, emotionally and in our lives in general.

Throughout the text we will never insist enough with regard to our health care as the fundamental premise for adopting intermittent fasting and the diets necessary for it. This book offers both information, tricks and methods to ensure the effectiveness of this new habit, as well as care and general advice scattered throughout these words to draw attention to the importance of having a systemic and holistic view of our body in order for us to identify which are the real problems that accompany us in our daily lives and how would be the best approach to begin to solve them.

If you consider this book to be an important tool for you and/or others who aim to improve their health, well-being and lives, above all, make sure to let us know what you liked most about the text, whether or not you would recommend it and share positive reviews about it, which is the result of extensive research and collective experiences with intermittent fasting.

The intermittent fast

It is a common misconception to assume that fasting is a form of diet and that it can be assumed indiscriminately. First of all, there are conceptual differences between what diet is and what fasting is. While the former refers to a set and to a number of meals that make up a person's diet, the latter is understood as deprivation of food consumption for a limited period of time. Diets include not only the dietary regimens that some of us assume with a rather clear goal in mind: weight loss, weight gain, muscle mass, definition, or simply an improvement in our quality of life. Diets also include those traditions, customs and habits that people have depending on various factors, especially those of a social, cultural and geographical nature, because depending on social interactions, from the culture to which they belong and from the environment from which they get the food, so the diet will also be influenced.

What interests us in this text is not so much the diet, but the fasting, the deprivation of food for a specific period. However, in a similar way to diet, it is advisable to consult professional help to determine the viability and fasting regimen that should be pursued in order to achieve our goal as well as to preserve and improve the condition/health of our body, Depending on the *background* of each person, their previous habits, previous and/or chronic health conditions, there will be different methods of application and adoption of fasting.

Continuing with the main idea, if fasting is the deprivation of food for a certain time, then it is logical to assume that the *added intermittency in the name of the method refers to a constant interruption of this fasting process. While this may become confusing because the science of fasting-or rather what our common sense tells us-is not to interrupt food deprivation, the truth is that the scheduled interruption of fasting under a few margins away from radicality promotes the benefits of this way of eating, of this eating habit, without going too far to promote the emergence or development of eating disorders known today as anorexia, to mention some example. In this sense, the intermittency of fasting is distributed on a daily basis; that is, we fast daily for a certain amount of hours that we must respect as a soldier in the army.*

Ideally, the amount of fasting hours set should be methodically adequate depending on the conditions of each person interested in adopting this habit, but generally speaking, It is common to find recommendations everywhere about maintaining a 12-12 fasting regimen, or what is the same, 12 hours of fasting and 12 hours of normal feeding. This must obviously respect the pace of life of each person as their adaptation must be consistent and realistic. As a general rule, the hours of sleep are also counted as hours of fasting, because in fact you do not find yourself ingesting any type of food. If the average sleeping hours comprise eight hours, it means that, in a waking state, or what we might call actual *fasting hours*, we would actually have to fulfill at will only four hours of fasting after waking up. For some people this could mean breakfast in the middle of the morning, directly waiting for lunch or lunch a little earlier than usual. Depending on the time we eat that will be equally proportional to the hours in which we do not eat but respect the fast.

On the other hand, several experts, while recognizing the benefits of having an intermittent fast under the 12-12 regimen, have found that a 16-8 fasting has generally delivered better results for people who have adopted that regimen. This means -again, in general terms- that we would have eight hours of fasting that comprise the hours of *sleep and then 8 actual* hours of fasting that establish the time of meal already well past lunch hours. Of course, this will depend on how each person manages their time. What, if we recommend at the beginning, for an easier adoption of this new habit, is that if you are a person who usually sleeps little by habit, this is a good opportunity to fix your sleep schedule.

The reasons for adopting intermittent fasting range from a way to help weight loss to a way to make your time more efficient and invest in the activities you most want to do. But if fasting is just a way/habit of eating, can you lose weight just by changing a habit? Without a doubt, many cases have been reported with positive results of weight loss, also having as another of its main benefits the reduction of anxiety to eat that many people, especially overweight, suffer. The question now seems to be directed to how intermittent fasting helps weight loss and control eating anxiety

The human body: a

perfect system

To start talking about how intermittent fasting helps us lose weight, it is necessary to first understand in general and abstract aspects how our body works internally and externally, and then understand it at more specific levels. In this sense, it is important and necessary to extract some of the contributions of the general theory of systems, mainly the contributions of the scientist Ludwig von Bertalanffy, who developed the theory from a biological point of view, the one that most interests us.

In general terms, the general theory of systems has fundamental premises which are that all biological systems are open systems and that they also exist in constant interaction with other systems. These interactions occur within an even larger system that contains them, in a permanent dynamic of interaction and exchange of matter and energy.

In simpler terms, this means that all systems, in order to survive, need to obtain vital resources from the environment to which they belong -ergo, other systems. In turn, these other systems that we feed on also need the input of other systems to sustain ourselves. Thus, the only way in which systems can exist and survive is under the idea that all parts of it must function properly so as not to affect the functioning of the system to which we refer, and this also includes the proper functioning of other systems from which one is directly or indirectly interdependent.

Why are we talking about systems? Surely we will have heard in our lives when referring to certain complex sets of our system: nervous system, digestive system, bone system, and so on. However, there seems to be a common belief-if you even get that idea-that the human body is made up of systems, without considering that the body itself is a system that constitutes others. The failed functioning of any of these body systems affects the functioning of the whole body either indirectly or indirectly. In the case of the human body, if the nervous system, considered the central system of all who make up the body, is affected, it is a fact that the whole of our body will have negative consequences, especially those related to consciousness and mind, as these are found directly in the brain, but it is important to remember that the brain also controls the functioning of the rest of the operations of the body by means of other elements and/or organs that serve as an appendix to them to be able to work according to the total functioning of the body. Examples of these "appendages" include the heart, kidney, livers, thyroid, among many others. Each of these extensions, designed and specialized to serve specific parts of the body, have an interdependent relationship with the whole body and with the brain. This relationship of interdependence explains why by failing some of these organs the human body is unable to operate properly and can sometimes lead to death. Other simpler ways of raising this question are simply asking the question: with what set of elements, organs, systems, can we not live? The various answers that may come out of this question always lead to a fundamental concept of the system vision of our body: the concept of synergy. Synergy is nothing more than the coordination of the various elements of the structure that make it function as a whole, it is the understanding that the totality of things is greater than the sums of their own parts. That is, the nervous, digestive and bone systems are nothing in themselves; are unable to function properly if the nervous system is not able to control the functions of the other systems; the digestive system to process energy inputs and distribute them to all parts of the body; and the bone system to nourish itself from this energy, sustain the body and protect its other systems to ensure its own functioning. Often the concept of synergy is summarized under the phrase: *the whole is greater than the sum of its parts*. To do so, each of its parts must function properly.

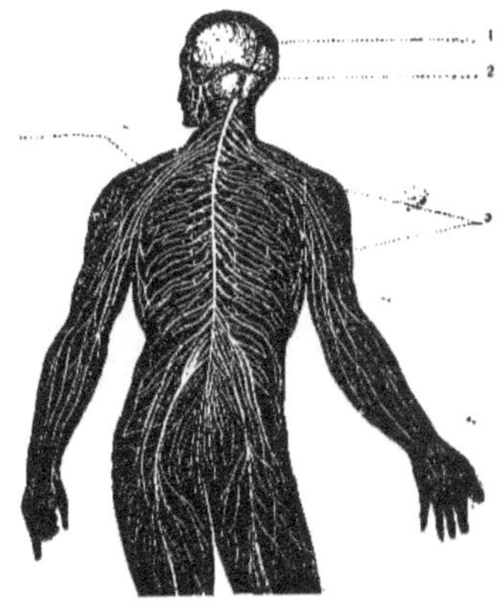

A system is a set of interrelations that cannot be understood without observing the totality.

Under this order of ideas, systems can be defined as a set of interdependent elements-which may also be other systems-that are in constant interaction and exchange with other systems in order to survive and remain in operation.

The general theory of systems indicates the existence of two types of systems: open systems and closed systems. Because we are talking about an organic system-we, the human body-have so far referred to an open system: open because it cannot live isolated from other systems, from its environment. We need nature, the different systems that exist in the ecosystem *in* order to exist: the rain, the pollination of flowers for oxygen, vegetables and animals -other organic systems- used in agriculture and livestock, among others.

What do systems have to do with fasting, specifically intermittent fasting? Organic, and thus open, systems operate in a certain way under a certain set of mechanisms according to the needs and capacities that the same system requires in its constitution: that is, they function depending on their structure and not outside of that structure. The mechanisms that make up the structure have a series of fundamental premises: maintaining the functioning of the system -in our case, living- the reduction or eradication of entropy levels, the assurance of the homeostatic process and the transformation of the inputs obtained by the feedback. Entropy refers to the levels of *chaos* or imbalance that can exist in our body-when we get sick, when we have nutritional deficiencies, etc.; the homeostasis process refers to the mechanisms that the body has to self-regulate its own functioning in the search for internal stability during the exchange with its environment -regulation of our temperature when we have fever, activation of the immune system, etc.; finally, the feedback uses some of the results of previous activities to relapse into other aspects of the body. Food, as one of the fundamental activities to keep our body alive, is a process of exchange with the environment: while the environment gives us food, the excrement that we expel as a result of food, although it is technically waste or waste from our body, it is an input to nature, specifically for plants:

in this case, we are talking about the feedback that exists between our body and plants, and that in turn refers to the process of neguentropy, which is nothing more than the expulsion of entropy -waste- from our body. As long as we feed, depending on how we feed and what we feed, our body will also be regulated to ensure its own functioning even if there are deficiencies in the material and energy inputs that we provide to it via our food: the body will do everything possible with the resources available. In this sense, intermittent fasting is a way to provide our body with the food supplies it needs in a more optimal and efficient way taking into consideration the environment in which our body is today. Thus, we take advantage of the homeostasis process and the neguentropy of our body to expel waste and regulate abnormalities in our body, such as excess fat and anxiety about eating.

Understanding our body as a system means understanding that food will irremediably affect our whole body beyond its figure, its shape and its weight: from our intelligence, emotions, to our performance in our work, in our hobbies, in the capacity of our system/body to, first, keep us alive, and second, make this life optimal.

For this reason it is that the consequences of a poor diet sustained for many years -and of anything else harmful to the health of our body- are not visible if not when it turns out to be too late, unless we talk about something extremely aggressive for us and the results are quickly visible, so that we can relate causes and effects almost immediately. This phenomenon is known as boiled frog syndrome.

The story tells how a frog jumps immediately upon being thrown into boiling water, but that if it is placed in water and then raised to a temperature until it slowly comes to a boil, it will be too late for the frog to react and it will die, as your body is not designed to detect progressive changes in your temperature

The boiled frog syndrome is an analogy concerning how the consequences of very slow harmful processes are not possible to make visible in the immediate reality, at present, and therefore go unnoticed or are deliberately ignored at the time because they are not considered relevant or of great impact until it is too late to act and try to solve it, as the damage is usually structural and can no longer be repaired.

This analogy refers to awareness of problems rather than knowledge of problems. It is known that a bad diet harms our body and our general well-being, but sometimes there is no awareness of these consequences because it is not possible to see them in the immediacy of our time and we dismiss them consciously or unconsciously, Even though we know for sure the seriousness of the facts. The same happens with habits, exercises, lifestyles, and a long etcetera.

Along the lines of this argument, it is important to identify not only the nutrients and foods we need during intermittent fasting in order to maintain our body in the best conditions available, but, in addition, it is necessary to determine the frequency with which we can ingest certain types of food -some are more beneficial to eat at certain times, every certain number of days; others are easier to digest and can be ingested more often, etc.-, knowing and being aware of what are the stages of the process, and how intermittent fasting interacts with other of our daily activities, with our performance in each of them, etc.

Effects of intermittent fasting on the body

The first thing the body perceives is a cut in its energy supply. This impact on the functionality of the body causes it to enter a state of homeostasis that, remember, is a process of regulation of every system that seeks to maintain stability in its functioning by providing energy to each of its parts: bones, muscles, organs, hormones, other systems, etc. In this case, seeing the supply of energy disappeared for the body, it begins to use the reserves that our body stores precisely for these situations. It does this quickly by sending a signal to our brain that we need to replenish energy and, in the absence of food, the brain coordinates with the whole body to start using all the fats, carbohydrates, glucose and so on to keep the body functioning. For this reason it is impossible to burn body fat at specific sites, such as in the abdomen, legs or even the neck, but it does so uniformly everywhere where there is excess fat and where it is more difficult to disappear it, is where it is most accumulated. For our body, the totality of its parts also serves as a great reservoir of energy.

If we are already clear on why our body begins to use stored energy in the form of excess fat, the next question to answer is when this process occurs.

The most important reason why fasts should be observed with discipline and strictness is that they are directly and closely related to the results of fasting. Without perceiving any food, the human body takes about twelve to fourteen hours to trigger alarms throughout the system and begin to use the stored energy. In this sense, then it would be appropriate to make a minimum fasting of between twelve or fourteen hours respectively (of course, this will always depend on the type of intermittent fasting that each person performs). This state of alarm -so to speak- in which the body enters to begin to burn its reserves is known as the process of ketosis. Like any process of alarm, these results from a response that the body exercises before the emergency of the deprivation of food and, therefore, of energy source. States of alarm, in general, are usually related to high levels of tension between the agents involved and affected by the situation that warrants the emergency. Thus, it is important to understand that prolonged states of alarm, while ultimately aiming to restore the balance of the body, can become risky because of the high loads of stress that the body is in a permanent state of emergency. Not only in the context of intermittent fasting, but also in any other type of excessive stress, such as physical, atrophied muscles, and mental, chronic anxiety.

Therefore, this homeostatic process, of self-regulation, has some important advantages and disadvantages to consider to make the most of while reducing the threats it may pose to health. Let's start by understanding ketosis well.

Ketosis: definition, advantages and disadvantages

As we have already mentioned in previous sections, the human body needs energy to maintain its functioning, energy that it subtracts from the environment by means of food and oxygen. However, not all energy comes from oxygen alone and not all food implies an energy contribution to its functioning. This explains why it is possible to see two people with the same weight and physical appearance and one of them has food deficiencies: one of them is not feeding her body well. This also explains why weight is not a determining factor in knowing a person's state of health. In addition, this also indicates that there is no single source of energy, which is why in diets that are considered balanced by experts around the world no matter what which context it belongs to, food diversity and variety is one of the decisive factors.

Sweets are a good example of those foods -or rather, things that we can ingest- that do not bring anything beneficial to our body -not even energy- and, on the contrary, what they do is actually increase the insulin in our body, threatening our health. On the other hand, eating only vegetables does not represent a good diet because it does not provide enough energy that the body needs to function and they are deprived of carbohydrates. At this point, what the body needs most as fuel are carbohydrates, its main source of energy. A deficit or deprivation of carbohydrates immediately translates into a reduction in the energy of our body and a physical and immune weakening, the functions of our body generally decrease: is what happens when we have a lot of time without eating and/or have not eaten anything until that specific time and we begin to feel these discomforts. Carbohydrates are an essential part of a healthy diet in any part of the world regardless of differentiating factors, such as culture and geography, as these constitute one of the essential macronutrients, container of vitamins and minerals necessary for human life and, therefore, our main caloric contribution.

But aren't calories an enemy of weight loss? What's the use of depriving my body of something it needs to live? If I want to lose fat, why should I eat fat? While carbohydrates are the main source of energy for our body, let's remember that what our body really needs are calories as fuel, which can also be found in the fat that we have stored in our body over time. This function also makes fat another macronutrient that contains the necessary inputs for our body, as with carbohydrates. The fundamental difference is that while carbohydrate is the main source of energy, which it uses in the possible immediacy, fat is the secondary source of energy, reserve energy. Under this logic, to keep the battery of our cell phones charged, the first thing we would do is look for a plug and connect the charger directly to that power source; if for various reasons we can not have a plug or we do not have access to it, we can choose to use a second battery, powerbank.

Failing that, allow the battery to be completely discharged or turn off the cell phone to save the remaining battery. At this point, it is counterintuitive to use a powerbank or second battery when we can have any plug (that's why we have the second battery, to start with). It's the same with our body; for him, it's counterintuitive to burn fat if he can eat carbohydrates. Unlike the cell phone, we cannot simply replace the battery -decide to burn fat instead of carbohydrates-, although we can turn off to save energy. But in the same way that a cell phone turned off with the battery on still consumes power, The same happens with our body when we are sleeping to maintain the vital functions of the body and to set in motion different processes and own of the state of sleep, very different from the processes that it carries out -at least at the mental level- when we are in a state of vigilance. It is important to note that the brain and body continue to function in the same way as when we are sleeping or awake, but in different states of activity.

The inherent inability to decide what kind of energy to use-whether carbohydrate or fat-, when to use it, and in which parts of the body corresponds to the systemic nature of our body: each of its parts is interdependent and all are affected if any of them are. For this reason, it is that the whole body must enter into a specific state in which it is forced to use the reserves of energy as primary sources of resources for itself; the whole body, then, must enter into a state of ketosis.

The state of ketosis refers to a metabolic situation in your body that, faced with the deficiency or total absence of carbohydrates, begins to use the energy reserves manifested in the form of fats. In other words, in the absence of carbohydrates, you burn fat. This is achieved by releasing ketones that break down your body's adipose tissue into essential nutrients. This process can also be accelerated if exercise routines are executed by the demand for energy to which the body will be subjected during the activity. However, it is important to emphasize that a deficit in carbohydrate intake should not mean a nutritional deficit; if so, rather than burning the body's fat it will begin to decompensate and degrade its functions. The ideal situation to take advantage of cetosis while accompanying it with exercise, is to identify and carry out a feeding plan that guarantees us the essential nutrients.

Accompanied by induction into a state of ketosis, some people have also opted for the ketogenic diet, which consists of reducing carbohydrate consumption between twenty and fifty grams per day. The reasons for adopting both a ketogenic diet and a food habit in the form of intermittent fasting are generally due to the fact that the benefits represented by the combination of the two methods offered similar results to the adoption of a prolonged fasting. However, not all about intermittent fasting and, above all, ketogenic diet is only beneficial, and there are some important disadvantages to consider to take care of our health and still continue to take advantage of the benefits of these new feeding methods. Thus, we can make the following evaluation of the pros and cons of intermittent fasting.

The Benefits of Intermittent Fasting

The first advantage that the state of ketosis represents is twofold: it allows to control the amount of insulin in the blood while favoring the increase of growth hormone in the muscles. This is because insulin, as the vehicle by which it supplies energy -and especially carbohydrates- to the rest of the body by means of transporters, favors the use of fat as energy and as a nutrient for muscle growth. Under this logic, in a state of ketosis it is beneficial to generate more muscle mass because it reduces the amount of fat in your body: instead of transporting carbohydrates to the parts that need energy as a result of exercise, use fat as a replacement. This is even more beneficial when we consider that fat is about three times larger in volume than muscle. That is, 5 kilos of fat are bigger and take up more space in our body-and therefore, makes us look fatter-than five kilos of muscle.

The improvement in insulin control and performance also results in an improvement in metabolic and cardiovascular health, as well as an increase in sports performance.

We have already mentioned another of the benefits: it is the flexibility with which we can handle this method in relation to the hours we assign to eat. Depending on the responsibilities of each person and age, sometimes it is even inconvenient to "skip" breakfast because we require training before work, or do some other activity that we can prioritize and that would normally be sabotaged or interrupted by breakfast. The flexibility in the schedule to eat is a great advantage when we can eat what we need when our daily life allows us and we do not try to force it within a few moments that are incompatible with our personal dynamics. This is especially true when there are people who, for example, do not wake up hungry and are "forced" to have breakfast without actually having the need to eat.

The distribution of frequencies and amounts of food is also a characteristic and beneficial factor for those who decide to adopt intermittent fasting. As a general rule, there is a common idea that there should be at least three large meals throughout the day: breakfast, lunch and dinner corresponding to the morning, noon and night. Some insert the snack as another meal. Others, especially those who want to accelerate metabolism, distribute the same amount of food divided between four or five meals throughout the day. That is, the same amount of food that would be consumed in the traditional distribution of three meals a day are rationed into four or five dishes a day.

One of the possibilities of intermittent fasting is that it allows you to make between two or three large meals sufficiently satisfactory to allow you to go through the hours of fasting much more easily without breaking the necessary intake. Some others, even more radical, prefer to eat a huge single dish with a huge amount of food with all the calories and nutrients they need for that day. The latter find it somewhat difficult at first to adopt fasting, but it is extremely useful to them to make the most of their time over the course of a day. Of course, it takes considerably longer to eat that one dish.

Another benefit of intermittent fasting, and this refers to the main reason why some millennial peoples adopted fasting as a tradition, is to promote detoxification of the body. There are people who adopt intermittent fasting just to feel healthier, not just to lose weight. This is because several experts have claimed that intermittent aid contributes to autophagy. This process called autophagy is a natural detoxification process that consists of discarding the aged or unusable cell particles of our body and then proceed to the renewal of the eliminated cells, replacing them with new cells and regenerating the body.

While autophagy is a natural process that our body does constantly without help or deliberate intervention on our part, The truth is that today there are foods highly processed or intervened in some way that have made them particularly toxic to our body. As these foods come with chemicals, excess hormones, are refined, among other factors, as a consequence of the need to meet the demand for food worldwide since the last century especially, Our body has not evolved at the same speed as our society has, and therefore does not yet possess the natural mechanisms optimized enough to deal with all these invading agents at the rate that is really needed. For this reason, it is important that we contribute to it deliberately. Any process and/or food we can use to promote the autophagy process will always be welcome and grateful in our body and in our health, always staying within a not excessive, appropriate margins.

Disadvantages and risks of intermittent fasting.

(fat) stored. One of the first disadvantages refers specifically to women who adopt this way of eating. This disadvantage has to do more with the natural design of the woman's body by default, as it is commonly believed that the woman's body is more susceptible to hormonal problems.

Without a doubt, intermittent fasting can negatively affect the hormonal balance because, being designed the body of the woman to procreate life, faced with the partial or total absence of the necessary inputs -carbohydrates, energy- this reacts with a defense mechanism that prevents or hinders for the most part the use of fat as a main source of energy, because the logic of its functioning tells the body that its procreative capacity, its fertility, must be safeguarded -and this also obviously includes "saving" the body. This defense mechanism, which works in both men and women, but which in women has a particular incidence, responds by secreting a hormone known as ghrelin, known mostly as the hunger hormone. This hormone is also responsible for the prominent accumulation of abdominal fat, and when activated as a result of prolonged fasting, it tells your stomach and your whole body that you should eat urgently: This is conducive to a particularly unusual appetite and is the reason why it is sometimes difficult to lose fat. Not only because your body is uncontrolled at the hormonal level and practically forces you to eat on impulse, but the rest of your body is also induced to preserve energy reserves (fat) One of the first disadvantages refers specifically to women who adopt this way of eating. This disadvantage has to do more with the natural design of the woman's body by default, as it is commonly believed that the woman's body is more susceptible to hormonal problems.

This does not at all mean that women cannot perform or adopt intermittent fasting. Of course, there are exceptional cases that do not suffer from any of these disadvantages, but because they are not the general normal, women must take special care.

The approach or strategy frequently used in these cases is in the gradual adoption of intermittent fasting. That is, instead of starting the first day of the week immediately with a regimen of sixteen hours of fasting and eight hours of eating, it is most appropriate to start with a twelve-hour fast: the minimum time. Once adopted for a time the 12-12 regimen, depending on the needs of people and also physical limitations, you can gradually increase the amount of fasting hours to, For example, 13-11, for as many weeks as necessary until the body gets used to it.

At this point we are already talking about taking advantage of the homeostatic-self-regulatory process of our body to adopt new forms of activity and new forms of life. Just as when we exercise, we can't wait to do the same repetitions and exercises as someone who has been doing it for years now, but we can do it with training, practice, discipline and dedication. The same applies in the case of intermittent fasting and is especially useful as a strategy for women's bodies to successfully adopt this new eating habit. This gradual adoption of intermittent fasting is done with two major goals in mind. First, that the body become progressively accustomed to a new dynamic and thus lessen the physiological and psychological difficulty of adopting a new habit; and second, to avoid triggering the alarms of our body by the sudden change in diet, In adapting to a new normality, the parameters or indicators under which the defence mechanisms are activated naturally are modified and adapted.

Macronutrients: carbohydrates and fat

To have a greater and better understanding of how intermittent fasting works, it becomes necessary to understand its main agents:

carbohydrates and fats. Contrary to popular belief, not all carbohydrates are good and not all fats are bad. Let's start with carbohydrates.

Carbohydrates, as we have already mentioned, are a macronutrient that contains a multitude of elements that are necessary for the body, so this first description should not be a warning sign for our purposes with intermittent fasting, whether to lose weight or feel healthier with a new eating habit. Carbohydrates can be easily identified on any plate when placed as a companion to the main meal.

Carbohydrates can be classified simply as good and bad;

more technically, as refined and whole. The first, refined carbohydrates, are what we should avoid to the extent of the possibilities, since they consist of sugars, white flours and most processed products that we can find in any supermarket or supply, like breads, cookies and soft drinks. The main disadvantage of refined carbohydrates is that they are extremely easy to assimilate by our body, increasing sugar levels. This is what causes when we consume a lot of sugar we feel tired quickly, and how it is not advisable to consume sugars drinks because, while it gives a small boost of energy, The fact is that the energy effect is too short and the fatigue you feel after the effects of sugar is even greater than before consuming it. This is the result of sugar being assimilated so quickly by the body, high levels of insulin are generated to transport these nutrients to all parts of the body, but this generates greater tiredness and greater appetite, So, if you are near the limit of your caloric or carbohydrate deficit, this will make the process even more difficult. On the other hand, whole carbohydrates are the most ideal for daily consumption in our diet. These include fruits, starches such as oats, pasta and potatoes, and fibrous carbohydrates, which are even more important, such as vegetables. The latter represent an important advantage because the fibrosity of the tissues of plant food increases the levels of satiety they cause in the body and, as a result, generates less urgency for eating. These foods also include an essential part of ketogenic diets, since they make it easy to respect the limit of 30-50 grams of carbohydrates per day for the net value they provide and allow to control the appetite for their satiety levels.

Carbohydrates containing high levels of fructose-fruit sugar-and starches should be consumed in moderation. This is because the sugars used in soft drinks especially are extracted from this component. In addition to studies that indicate that consuming this element in large quantities is what generates the problems of obesity and diabetes. In context, in what refined carbohydrates like the aforementioned pages are characterized, is that they have very high concentrations of this sugar contained in quantities not equally proportional, but smaller. To give an example with fictitious values, if an average whole fruit provides 50g of sugar, half of that same fruit would have about 300g of sugar if it were a soft drink. Thus, due to the ease of assimilation of these sugars -which generates tiredness and arouses appetite- and the few amounts of food with high concentrations -plus assimilation of greater amounts of sugar, more appetite, more tiredness Over-consumption not only sabotages attempts at any specific healthy diet and intermittent fasting, but also poses a serious health risk.

Similar to carbohydrates, there are good fats and bad fats; more technically, processed/transaturated fats and natural fats. The former are frequently manufactured by man, are artificial to some extent and do not have any type of nutritional contribution to our body; the latter, as is obviously done, come directly from organic and natural sources.

Just like anything else, excess is harmful to our health, including fats. However, there are people who sometimes have more fat phobia than carbohydrates, especially when fat is present in the natural oils with which we usually prepare our food. While excess fat is harmful to health- for example, fried foods are a good way to represent this excess-there are people who are extremely thorough with the use of these oils, and others who prefer not to use them at all to eradicate the consumption of natural fats. This behavior has some validity, while food dripping oil is more harmful than anything else, but it is also necessary to consider that cooking oils are mainly used to promote the cooking of food as its digestion. This justifies why many people choose, for example, to buy the most natural and pure oil they can find-often olive oil- and add it, for example, to salads and some meats. In these cases, we consider it important to know the usefulness of certain resources-food, in some way, are also resources-and to use them with the necessary prudence to always make the most of them while diminishing the threats they pose to our bodies. In the case of natural fats, oils, if a product already has its own sufficient fat then we advise to use it for cooking without adding additional oils; on the other hand, if there are foods with which you have problems or difficulties to digest, Adding a little natural oil will help your assimilation.

What other ways are there to deal with the carbohydrate wall?

As we already know at this point in the reading, the main difference between carbohydrates and fat is that the first is the body's main source of energy; the second is the backup of this main energy.

The options available are no secret today in the information age. The most practical and traditional ways to break down the carbohydrate wall are, first, to enter a caloric deficit. Calorie deficit is to reduce your daily calorie intake below your usual calorie intake, preferably relative to the calories your body, depending on your weight, height, age, and gender, needs. That is: if a person of 25 years who measures 1.63 m, whose appropriate weight should be 55 kg and his current weight is around 80kg, this means that there is an excess in the caloric intake: this person consumes appropriately 3000 calories daily. If your body, with these characteristics, requires 2500 calories to function properly without becoming overweight, it means that it has an excess calorie of 500g. In order to enter a calorie deficit, the person should begin to reduce his caloric intake from 3000 calories to, ideally, about 2300. With this intake restricted below normal for your body, your body will begin to use those extra calories it has been accumulating over time in the form of fat. That is: start burning fat. However, this also depends not only on the natural caloric demand of your body, but also on the caloric demand demanded by the daily or particular activities of people in their daily lives. For example, a marathoner with a body with the same characteristics as mentioned above without being overweight, would need -by throwing fictitious values- around 5000 calories to be able to perform properly, without this meaning gaining weight or gaining weight, because the 5000 calories are being consumed in their entirety to make the body function and to run the marathon. This means that the person uses so much energy, so many caloric resources, that he exhausts both the carbohydrates and the fats he consumes: he uses everything he eats.

That logic also applies to intermittent fasting, but not necessarily so. Caloric restriction in fasting hours can promote fat burning, yes, but people can also consume the same calories as always in a shorter period of time. This means that, if a person requires 2500 calories a day, with intermittent fasting, they may decide to consume them over 12 hours run on a 12-12 regimen, or consume those same calories within 8 hours on a 16-8 regimen. This is the main reason why it is often insisted that fasting is not a diet, but a habit, a way of eating. A person can adopt intermittent fasting even if his diet consists only of processed, refined and saturated fats and sugars; this is done either by accident or because he believes that, to compensate for poor nutrition, is constantly detoxifying your body. What actually happens in the medium and long term, even in short terms, is the aforementioned gradual and progressive decompensation of the body, not to mention the problem of perspective that is suffering from the boiled frog syndrome. A diet based on the above components is not sustainable and can easily lead to food deficits. Just remember the way sugars and insulin interact to begin to understand that after burning carbohydrates and fats, you begin to "burn" your muscles.

This is another opportunity to make the emphasis always need to consult professional help to make the best decision and draw the best possible plan for your body, for you and for your lifestyle. It is important to assess our current situation in order to design a strategy that will allow us to reach the goal. ¡ We don't want to end up with diabetes!

General Tips

With the considerations outlined in the previous chapter, it is sufficiently clear that diet and fasting can become totally independent of each other, which one does not necessarily imply the other. However, the communion between diet and fasting is a powerful combination to improve the effects of intermittent fasting and improve the state of ketosis, if your goal with fasting and diet turns out to be weight loss or burning excess fat from your body. The most mentioned combination refers to the restriction or decrease of carbohydrate intake, although it is not a determining factor in the success of intermittent fasting. It is important to remember that the main purpose for which intermittent fasting was thought is about the healthy benefits for the body, and it is also good to remember that maintaining excessive restrictions over excessive periods of time also results in a harmful spectrum of intermittent fasting.

In this order of ideas, the first recommendation we suggest is the effective control of portions of food. With regard to diets and intermittent fasting, with control we refer not only to the deliberate behaviour of planning and administering the food we consume for a particular purpose, but also knowing what is going on as we put our plan in motion, whether they are positive or negative things of our performance in this new eating style; if we know the things we are doing well, This gives us an opportunity to modify our plan to improve our consumption or, on the other hand, to give us the satisfaction and confidence to be able to persist in this new activity in case it is difficult at the motivational level. In other words, the control of our activity is the first and fundamental step in evaluating our performance.

The question would be, now, how do we do it? Digital scales are a frequently used tool to maintain a thorough control over the amounts of calories we are consuming. If we get information about how many calories are in the different foods that we consume based on how many grams of those same foods, we will have the ability to determine with sufficient precision the amount of grams we need to consume daily to stay within the caloric deficit. If we have a body that weighs 75 kilos, this means that, on average, we need to consume 60 grams of protein and 1800 calories per day to stay healthy and in calorie deficit. If in our dish of the day we decide to eat lentils, these have 9 grams of protein and 115 calories per 100 grams of lentil that we are going to eat. This means that we should consume around 700 grams of lentils daily to meet our body's demand for protein, which would also be equivalent to 800 calories out of a total of 1800 daily -I understand this last value as necessary to enter a caloric deficit. Of course, it is important to remember that variety is a fundamental part of any healthy diet, and that what is exposed here with lentils is just one example. Using the same logic and the same tool, we can control, organize and administer all types of food based on the nutrients they possess for each certain amount of grams/weight. If we know the nutritional value per gram of food, it is enough to calculate and distribute over a day the amount of grams, nutrients and proteins we need to stay healthy.

However, without this tool Sometimes it is difficult and even desperate not to know if what we are consuming corresponds to what is necessary to achieve our goal or if we are even wrong, regardless of the reasons why a digital scale or similar tool for weighing food cannot be obtained. Thus, another way to have an approximate control of the quality and quantity of food we consume is to administer the foods by portions. For this is not necessary any specific tool or instrument, as we will only need our dish that we use to eat. With this dish, we are going to draw an imaginary line that allows us to divide it into several parts. We will begin by dividing the plate in half and in one of these halves we will place our vegetables; we will proceed by dividing the other half that is empty into two other halves, corresponding to two quarters of the plate; in each of these smaller halves, From these quarters, we will place a portion of protein and/or fat and a portion of carbohydrates respectively.

Among the particular methods similar to that of the plate, but not so usual we have that of the use of the hand. Basically, it consists of administering portions of your plate according to specific positions of your hand: the proteins must be equivalent to the size of the palm of your hand, the vegetables equal to two palms of open hands and together, sugars and oils are measured by reference to the tip of a thumb, the size of the fruit corresponds to your clenched fist.

These particular methods lack the high precision provided by the digital scale, and although they may seem like methods we would learn from our grandparents, always have some truth and effectiveness which is what has allowed them to remain throughout time as effective techniques or methods. For this reason, more rustic methods can provide effectiveness, although if we are a little doubtful about it, we can always rely on the advantages of the balance.

Now, we already have the general recommendations regarding the possibilities, tools and techniques that can help you to have better control, organization and administration of your diet while you adopt intermittent fasting. It is also useful to know what are the limits that break or impair the effectiveness of our fasting period, which we have not yet defined.

In spite of all the information that we have presented in this text, and of the large amount of information that can be found these days on the internet, progressively, there are still people who believe that they can eat in periods of fasting. Just to clarify, although we have defined fasting as a eating habit, it is necessary to spend at least 12 to 16 hours without eating any food, at all, for its effectiveness. It is necessary to remember that fasting is literally to stop eating for a certain period of time.

The best ally of intermittent fasting: water

Water is the first known source of life in our universe. It is from where the first unicellular beings originated and where the first advances of much more complex organisms manifested. It is not in vain that on other planets in our universe, where this liquid water does not exist, there is no life at all. The importance of water is such that the body can last several weeks without consuming any type of food, which is totally different with the consumption of water: in a matter of days the body deprived of vital liquid will begin to decompensate faster than if deprived of food.

The many benefits of water range from supporting the body's detoxification through urine and sweating-acting as a totally natural purifying agent and helps reduce the impact on our body when you are tired and begin to suffer fatigue. It also promotes the prevention of constipation, improving the digestive processes of our body and, last but not least, contributes to the elimination of by-products of fat that are in our body, especially when we're talking about artificial components.

Some experts suggest that the appropriate amounts of water vary depending on each person's body weight in water. Some people may wonder what body weight in water is and/or how they can get to know it. This is really simple to know: each liter of water equals one kilo of our weight. If we hold a container that can hold up to two liters of water, the container will immediately weigh about two kilos more than the container can weigh in a certain way. The next thing we need to know is the amount of water our bodies naturally possess; according to experts, the amount of water varies depending on sex and height, but the proportions are naturally the same. This means that about 60% of the body weight in men and 50% of the body weight in women is water. That is to say, if a woman weighs around 80 kg, it is right to presume that at least 40kg of her entire weight corresponds to her weight in water: we are talking about there being at least 40 litres of water in the body of a woman weighing approximately 80kg. Other information also suggests that the amount of water to be consumed daily varies greatly from the environment in which our body is located and from the activities to which we subject it. Among the factors that influence the amount of water our body needs to replenish is both physical activity, age, sex, body temperature and surrounding temperatures. Thus, the popular belief that at least six to eight glasses of water should be consumed daily is more a kind of myth than a reality according to some other experts. In these cases, what they most recommend is something quite simple: drink water when we are thirsty, consider thirst as if it were hunger or tiredness, because it is when we enter these states that the body tells us directly that we need to drink water, eat or sleep, respectively. However, it is not that drinking six or eight glasses of water a day does not have any benefit, as they state that if you want to eliminate extra calories, constantly going to the bathroom can help this purpose. Finally, they also recommend not going to the other end of the scale. That is, drinking too much water; there are cases of athletes who, without any scientific evidence or truly professional assistance, have been hospitalized for drinking too much water and some have even lost their lives. This is because the excess water dilutes the sodium found in our blood which results in an inflammation of our brain and lungs as a response to the organism trying to execute the homeostatic process -self-regulation- and levelling blood sodium levels to the best of their ability, which can lead to cardiac arrest. This is why when a person is admitted to a hospital for dehydration or some general decompensation of the body, doctors give electrolytes to our body and not water directly, Because electrolytes are the ones that really help regulate the behavior of our organism. A deficiency in electrolytes can often result in cramps in the body when we do some physical activity; in more important cases, which are not at all common, is when the body is cramped and no physical activity is being done. In these cases, we advise to see a doctor as soon as possible to determine the causes.

Continuing with electrolytes, these should be considered similar to how we treat the other nutrients in our body, such as proteins, carbohydrates, and calories, because there is a general consensus that electrolytes are considered to be the oil that lubricates the entire body for its operation. For this, it must be understood that there are several electrolytes, and that the electrolytes themselves are a compound of components: sodium, magnesium, calcium, potassium and chlorine. These components can be found in many unprocessed, organic-natural foods, such as fruits and vegetables, such as avocados, bananas, dried fruits, spinach, among others.

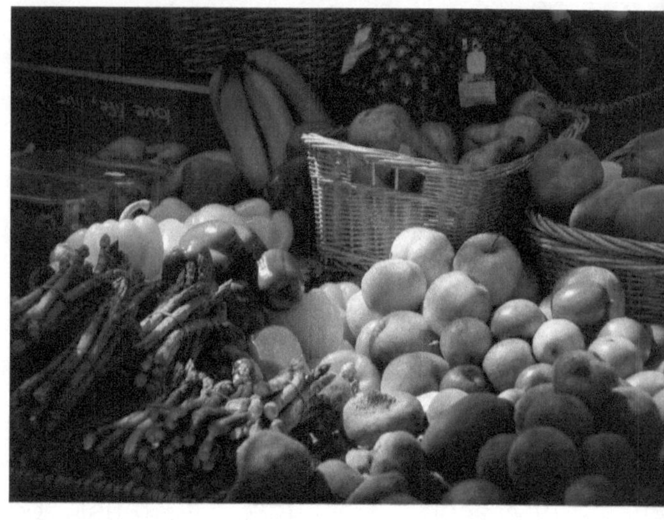

Variety is always an indispensable factor in any diet that is considered healthy.

Before and after: contrast of our eating habits

- We will start this chapter with a big question: how do you eat normally? Some of you may not have even thought for a moment about what your current eating habits are and what diet you have been following so far, and for how long. The truth is that few people really consider this situation and simply focus on making the qualitative leap of their food life. Everyone will have their own particular reasons why this happens, among those already known as the daily hustle and bustle or the dynamics of life at a personal level. Despite these particularities, it is important to ask ourselves this question in order to understand from where we are going to leave and where we are going to go: This will allow us to formulate all the necessary strategies and use the tricks or psychological traps to make life easier in the adoption of intermittent fasting as a kind of lifestyle.

-

- This question requires precision in a number of respects. From the content of our meals on a daily basis, such as the frequency at which we eat, the quantities, shapes, schedules, presentations of such food, and its origin, of course. Each of these elements that make up the question "how am I eating?" allow us to visualize more clearly what our feeding routine is.

-

- The most common and traditional food routine, which we also see in all the media, consists of:

-

- Get up early in the morning around or before eight or nine in the morning, where we will have our first breakfast consisting of carbohydrates, fruits or some protein, with the egg being the most usual presentation, accompanied as natural fats such as bacon or butter, depending on the culture, of the country.

*

* Throughout that same morning, it is common for people to prepare a drink to "accompany" their routine, being this drink in most cases coffee, tea or some type of juice/fruit juice.

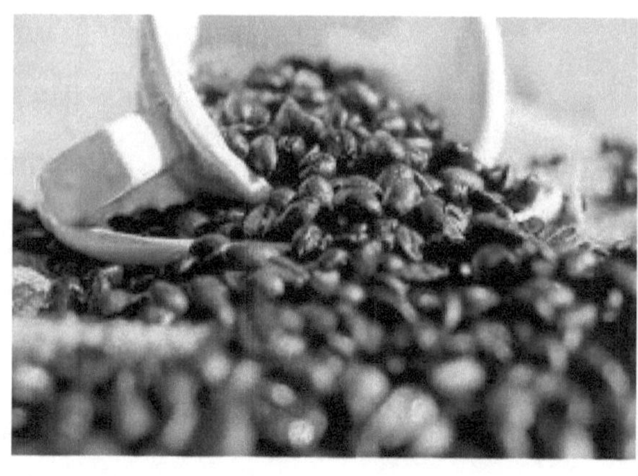

Coffee is one of the antioxidant drinks par excellence. Drink it in the mornings in periods of fasting favors and stimulate the digestive system.

- Then, between noon and the beginning of the afternoon, people proceed to eat lunch, food that is usually considerably larger in volume, much more substantial, and that usually contains processed carbohydrate foods and high levels of animal protein, perhaps accompanied by some vegetables.

*

* In the course of the afternoon many people generate craving for something sweet. Some go directly to consume sweets and other processed products, while others, more careful, opt for fruits or, failing that, nuts.

-

- By nightfall, people usually eat something similar to lunch, in terms of carbohydrates with protein, or directly repeat what they had for breakfast.

-

- Sometimes cravings can also wake up as late at night, similar to snack.

The first obvious observation of this process that we have described is that people who have adopted this habit either by tradition, accident or deliberately, are finding themselves eating at every moment of the day. By this we do not mean that eating is precisely a bad thing; on the contrary, our position has always been to defend healthy eating habits. What we mean is that the body is constantly on alert by digesting and assimilating food that we are sending to it, approximately every 2-3 hours. This pattern of feeding, this habit, progressively the body begins to get used to a very particular way of eating: if you get used to eating what is just and necessary, at first it will be difficult and then it will be easier for you to bear this burden; If you get used to eating bizarre amounts of food, you will gradually adapt to absorbing them.

This adaptation through which the body passes is based on artificial conditions that we have created for it. The fact that we give food to the body when it is not really telling us that it is hungry -because it really does not have it- makes us gradually deceive it, making it believe that every two or three hours it must be prepared to eat something. Getting used to this dynamic makes the body program itself as a kind of biological clock in which, even if you're not really hungry, it secretes the hormones that arouse the habit/appetite every two or three hours, and that's what the urge to eat usually generates. It is here that the main reason why diets are often complicated in the beginning, because it is about forcing the body to acquire new habits, it is about breaking their expectations regarding what hours and what will eat, which adds difficulty levels. This deceptive habit to our body easily results in a vicious circle and getting out of it results in a naturally slow process compared to our expectations of what we would really like, so consistency and discipline are important.

The above description is just a reference to the point that we must identify our feeding routine to get going and implement the relevant improvements. Once we understand our own routine, we can easily begin to point out the differences of these and what intermittent fasting involves.

As we already know, the main characteristic of intermittent fasting is the long periods of time in which we deprive ourselves of eating food, so naturally, when beginners start this activity, the first question that will be asked will be: How can I stand this long without eating? We already know that half of the challenge we overcome when we are sleeping the corresponding 8 hours out of a total of 16; if you are a person with not so healthy sleep habits, this can become a good trick to overcome the difficulty of fasting and, By the way, you reconcile your differences with sleep! Now there's only the other half, 8 hours left. What do we do?

Not all people wake up in the morning with an appetite but after a couple of hours of waking up. If you're one of the people who doesn't like breakfast or are indifferent to breakfast, you're in luck! If, on the other hand, you belong to that group that is used to breakfast and find it difficult to skip that meal, let's not panic! In these cases, the water will always be your faithful friend, because drinking it in good quantities favors the feeling of satiety in the stomach and will allow to control the feeling of hunger, but only temporarily. How long is it? It will depend on how much water you consume and how much appetite you have at that time, but in general, the vital liquid allows us to stretch our resistance in the hours of fasting and is a great ally in the first moments. Of course, we will not consume 10 liters of water as "breakfast" to withstand hunger: let us remember the risks of consuming excess water! Another trick we can take advantage of is to drink coffee or natural tea without any sugars: if it has sugar or is added to them, you lose automatically, because sugar will automatically activate our daily process of energy use.

In our intermittent fasting, we will usually start eating at about one or two in the afternoon, approximately -of course, it will depend on your schedule needs. The most recommended for the first meal of the day is to be as light as possible while providing all the nutrients we need, It is important to remember that our stomach comes from a fairly long period of fasting and is sensitive to anything we throw at it. Eating a heavy food as the first meal of the day is what usually causes inflammation, drowsiness and a generalized lethargy throughout the body, because all the energies of our body are focused on digestion (This is another reason why it is not advisable to shower after bathing! The body must allocate energy to maintain the body temperature while showering, and we just finished eating, the body will have to distribute that same energy to heat our body and do the digestion simultaneously, so neither process will do it in the most effective way possible and can even cause indigestion).

Another important recommendation is to focus on food while eating. Apart from distractions that do not favor digestion and proper chewing of food, we may fall into the error of consuming more than we should. Worse still, distracted eating contributes to lower satiety levels after eating, so it favors the appearance of appetite earlier than expected. In other words, if you eat distracted, you will be less satiated; if you concentrate on eating, you will be more satiated. We also recommend only eating until you are satiated and nothing else; taking into account that you have served more food than you are supposed to eat, or there are leftovers even after you have administered it correctly.

Once the afternoon passes, usually at five in the afternoon, it is valid to eat some fruit or a snack.

Finally, we have dinner. If you imagine that because dinner is necessary to eat something also light, we can say that we are a little wrong. It is important and necessary for our fast that dinner be a fairly substantial meal, because dinner is the last meal of the day until the middle of the next day. Sounds pretty loud, doesn't it? If we assume your dinner would be around seven and eight at night, it means you couldn't eat until one in the afternoon the next day. With so much time without food, the decision to eat substantial amounts of food at dinner is starting to make more sense. Because, although the hours of sleep count as fasting and is a great bridge to withstand the hours we should not eat, we have to make the remaining hours we have to be as manageable as possible. Again, you have to be careful not to exceed the amount of food or the amount of calories you need to consume, if you have adopted a ketogenic diet.

As we can see so far, the main difficulty in adopting intermittent fasting is a mental issue, where the cycles of anxiety originate and where the discipline we have to achieve our goals is manifested, or not. What we recommend, in simple terms, is to persevere long enough for the mind to get used to the changes that we naturally oppose, either consciously or unconsciously.

For example, it's normal for us to start counting every minute that goes by in the hours you can eat or can't eat, which creates a certain mental and body stress burden. Once you get used to it, this mental process sometimes stops being conscious and becomes an automatic behavior integrated into your own everyday life, so you don't need to think about it all day every day. Experts in different disciplines that have to do with the adoption of new habits -in subjects that include not only fasting and diets, but also in the area of psychology- they say almost in unison that letting go of old habits is often the most painful part of the whole process, occasionally through the process of dopamine detoxification, which we will discuss later. Therefore, the first few weeks are usually the most difficult and progressively the difficulty will be reduced as long as we maintain discipline and constancy in doing what we are supposed to do.

The mental dimension

It is often difficult-if not rare and almost exotic-to find the implications of everything concerning the mind with fasting and any dietary process.

Generally when we seek information regarding fasting and diets, we are always spoken of from the particular specialty that speaks about health, the body, the organism in general as a biological system. There are many times when the mind is not considered as part of the body and therefore has little to do with what happens to the mind and the impact it has on the body, or how the body has an impact with what happens in the mind. Information on the latter aspect is often easily identified and revolves around NGOs or organizations that seek to work to overcome inequalities and poverty in the world, but little consideration is given to the same aspects of information that people from more developed countries have even easier access to. This is a particular phenomenon because even though the data indicate that the developed *countries have the highest rates of patients suffering from mental illness or conditions -with higher rates of suicides compared to the poorest countries in the world-are the ones that least interrelate the knowledge of all scientific disciplines, including health disciplines, to improve the well-being of people. Under this logic, it makes sense for there to be infinite tons of information regarding fasting and dieting and little or no evidence of an intrinsic relationship with mental health, except sometimes, when only clinical conditions and conditions known as anorexia and bulimia are discussed. However, to get to the point of suffering some of these disorders there must be a process that has to be executed for a* certain time. That is, some of these disorders do not appear spontaneously, they do not appear out of nowhere; they are the product of a degenerative process in the mental health of some of the people that can last years. As a process, it means that it is a condition that needs to develop in order for the first symptoms or characteristics of these conditions to appear. However, it is not necessary to wait for diseases to appear to work on them; the best thing we can do is to prevent them with knowledge. For this reason, we consider it necessary to speak also of mental health, which is part of our body, without which our body could not operate and vice versa; always having in mind the systemic vision of *what we human beings are, body and mind are part of the same and complement each other, generate synergy.*

The unobserved obstacle: dopamine

At this point in the text we already know that some people do not necessarily wake up hungry immediately after opening their eyes. It is common for hunger to begin to appear once about an hour or two passes, depending on the person. At this point, if you wake up without an appetite, it's best to prolong that state of satiety as much as possible by staying away from everything that has to do with food. Focusing on particular activities can help put your focus on the activity and make your mornings a little more productive. Of course, this turns out to be the ideal scenario and not everyone necessarily has-or can-reach it. In addition, the advice to stay away from everything that has to do with food is incredibly valuable: if you are one of those people who follow many restaurants on their social networks and ask for delivery services constantly, these are your main enemies. Beyond the obvious causes, the ease of being able to access your favorite food with just a couple of clicks results in a kind of narcotic for your brain: the brain is loose by nature and will always look for the most convenient. The fact that fasting represents a period of some level of difficulty for our body, is because the brain dictates it, so it will naturally secrete the hormones of appetite so that you take it out of that state of "suffering". If you add to this the fact that you have the facility to access your favorite food with a couple of clicks and without even cooking it, the brain will naturally betray your consciousness -and your body-making it believe that it has the urge to buy food through delivery services, because it is tasty and does not require too much effort, besides that you are hungry!

Fighting the brain is sometimes a struggle in vain and unnecessary: in vain because we will often lose this fight, and unnecessary because there are better ways -smarter, sometimes even less effort- to control our behavior at will. For this reason, it is necessary to create conditions in our environment that will facilitate the fulfilment of our objective or, on the contrary, that will hinder our deviation from the objective, our own sabotage. In this sense, again, it becomes imperative to eliminate all types of access to any type of information that has to do with food: dishes, restaurants, recipes, promotions, and so on. Distancing ourselves from all content will not only be an advantage for the fulfillment of your intermittent fast, but, in addition, it will allow your brain to progressively regulate its dopamine levels generated both by the viewing of this content and by the consumption that these contents promote. For obvious reasons, if we have a refrigerator at our fingertips most of the time, put it in a place that makes it harder for you to access!

Now, what is dopamine? The technical and easily identifiable definition is that it is a neurotransmitter: this means that it is a kind of chemical/hormone that is generated in our brain. It is one of the main hormones responsible for regulating our emotions and that leads us to the pursuit of pleasure - and in some way, happiness- regardless of the type of pleasure that this is: sexual, sports, personal, professional, academic, etc. The variety of these stimuli depends on the bidirectional relationship we have with reality. First, it depends on what things mean to us at a certain point in our lives-eating hamburgers as a sort of post-workday ritual, for example-; second, the influence that things have on our perception, our sensations and our brains -addictive foods or drinks, the levels of pleasure they generate in our body both by consumable products and various activities.

The role that dopamine plays in this situation is that it incites -both the brain and you- the need to repeat that experience that generates a state of happiness/pleasure. The segregation of this hormone makes us motivated to get the necessary means to repeat such activity; for this reason is that addictions are difficult to overcome, because it is a problem that is found, in part, located in our brain and how our brain reacts to the stimulus, and what that stimulus means to us. The spectrum of addictions ranges from drug addiction to television addiction, to pornography and, of course, to some kind of food, especially sweets.

Because this variety of elements represents for our brain the ideal state of pleasure and happiness, when we begin to restrict what feeds our dopamine, The brain secretes a staggering amount of this hormone that makes us crave the things that give us pleasure. This is what is today known as that anxiety to eat, manifested especially in the consumption of sweets or sweets of any kind, as it is public knowledge that sugar has addictive components against which our brain is especially vulnerable. In other words, when this hormone is secreted in certain amounts in our brain, not only does it create anxiety about wanting to achieve that which gives us pleasure, but, on the other hand, it also generates an expectation: that yearning memory of pleasure that our brain so much seeks to repeat. When the brain does not meet that expectation generated by dopamine, it falls into a sort of depressive state, and this is a natural response of the organism. It is probably rare to hear a person get sad or depressed because he or she has entered a diet or started a fast, and this has its raison d'être in part.

In the case of food, as it is a primary and fundamental source to keep our body functioning, the brain does not hesitate or waste time in making us feel sad or happy when we are hungry or satiate it after a long period of fasting; What matters to the brain is somehow getting the food we need. This state of emergency usually leaves no room for emotions and simply triggers our instincts to look for food. This is perfectly natural, it is not abnormal; neither is the fact that we get depressed. It is a fact that some people have a particular relationship with food, to the point that they are substitutes for some kind of addiction. That's right, people can be addicted to food, even if this is our main source of life.

If we put ourselves in a situation where we're not addicted to food, but if we have some kind of relationship, "special with her, then it's no wonder we get sad or depressed because we're deprived of the types of food and ways of eating that we're used to. In other words, while the natural and instinctive response to food deprivation is the activation of hunger and the search for food, depression can also become a valid and perfectly natural response, depending on how we relate to food.

In the first case, the problem goes away when two things happen: we resist the urge to eat enough so that the body gets used to fasting and/or the new diet, or we just eat and satisfy our hunger, although this is not what we really want, right? In the second case -in which we get depressed- we go through a process of similar adaptation, because the hormones and chemicals of our brain and our body are crazy and unbalanced in the absence of the stimulus that generates pleasure, in the face of failure to meet expectations. Does this mean you're going to be depressed for life? Not at all. As in the first case -and recalling what we talked about understanding our body as a system- there are self-regulatory mechanisms that seek to restore the balance of our body to normal levels of functioning, even if this means establishing a new form of normal operation. This means that, in the absence of pleasurable stimulus and our brain possessing high levels of dopamine that are not being satisfied, we enter a depressive state as a natural response and, to return to a normal emotional state, the body over the days will seek to regulate the hormone levels of dopamine as long as we do not make the mistake of "satisfying" it, because that means you return to the state before the adoption of intermittent fasting and/or new diet.

In general terms, if you are one of the people whose organism responds by inducing you to a depressive state in front of fasting and the new diet; hold on! It is a natural response of your body and the most difficult part is in the first days -the first week according to some experts- because the body is just assimilating the new situation and the process of hormonal self-regulation is just beginning. After these first few days, you will see that you will feel better emotionally, that mood will be reduced or completely gone, and you will even begin to feel better than before you started fasting/dieting. It's all about consistency and discipline.

Anxiety and its possible causes

Anxiety is a highly prevalent psychiatric disorder today, especially in developed countries. It is characterized because people who suffer from it suffer from constant worries and periods of stress/distress without necessarily having a reason or cause of apparent origin. This does not mean that any moment of stress or concern means that we are already suffering from a psychiatric disorder; these states are part of our daily life and our naturalness as living beings because they are mechanisms that we have developed throughout our evolution to ensure our survival as a species.

In the case of stress and worry, experts say they can be classified into two types of stress; the one that paralyzes you and prevents you from doing something about it -bad stress- and the one that drives you and generates the necessary energies to enter a state of high concentration and performance of the activity you are performing -good stress. Stress and worry become a pathology when they occur with high frequency in a person's life, when it represents about half of the time in which the person is in a waking state and,

Above all, he begins to interfere with the activities of his own life. When these extremes begin to recur, it is when a person is usually considered to have anxiety. The diagnosis of any type of condition, especially of mental condition, always has to be endorsed by a health professional. This is meant to serve as a guide to clues that can help you identify a problem and proceed as best as possible with relevant assistance.

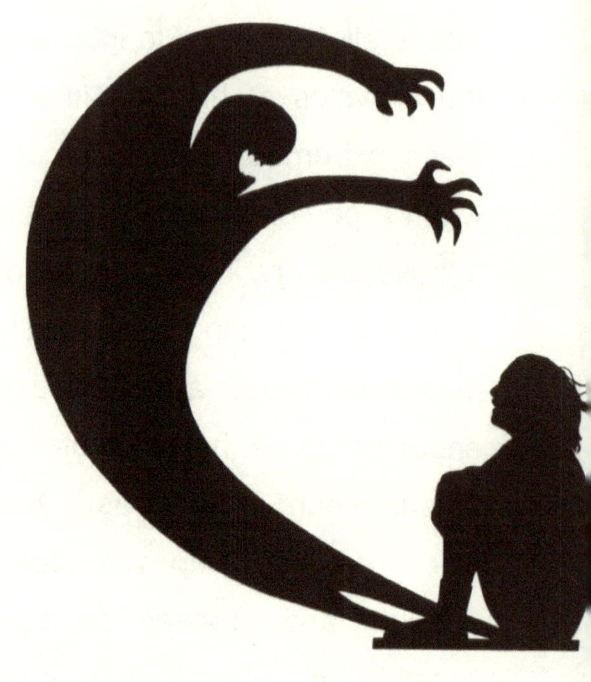

Anxiety is a natural reaction of our body

against what we may consider adverse or

dangerous

The origins of anxiety disorder are very heterogeneous due to the systemic nature of our body. We can refer from hormonal problems to the consequences of some past trauma. Pathological anxiety is characterized, as we mentioned, in that it begins to interfere with your own life and the way you carry on your daily life; it can affect your decision making, causing you to make decisions that you would not normally make or, on the contrary, stop.

Anxiety is usually manifested in the form of addiction, the most frequent being drug addiction-alcohol and so on-and food addiction. Although drugs can induce states of anxiety, in the case of food-unless it is specially prepared to be addictive-what is really the problem is the relationship that the person may have with food, conditioned by pathological anxiety. That is, food is not the bad thing, the bad thing is the relationship that the anxious person can have with food, which could lead to other pathologies and eating disorders such as obesity and anorexia, to cite some examples. These latter two disorders are also the most frequent manifestations of food anxiety; in the case of obesity, we see that they are people who overeat foods rich in sugars or very salty; At the other extreme, we have people who are kind of terrified of eating any kind of food, trying to ignore the clear signs of their body screaming that they are hungry. In both cases, the consequences may or may not be known to anxious people, but that does not come into the equation precisely because of the pathological condition of anxiety they suffer.

In the case of people whose anxious response is to eat a lot of food, this will also depend in part on what a lot of food is for that person or not. This has a direct impact on the amount of food that people eat and it also depends, of course, the levels of anxiety that manifest in your mind. It is above all by this last factor, that the person will feel more need to eat bizarre amounts of food, also known as binge eating, because his mind makes him believe that is the way in which he can satiate the discomfort that anxiety causes him, although we already know that this has to do more than anything with the role of dopamine in the whole hormonal and psychological, although not necessarily determinant and a professional diagnosis is the most prudent step to take.

One of the great difficulties of this type of problem, which are characterized by having a strong influence on our behavior, is that we are not aware of them in most cases. Many people are not aware of this almost impulsive feeding behavior and sometimes even are not able to notice it despite seeing the physical evidence: the changes and deterioration of their body and their health. The problem is further aggravated when they are so used to deteriorating health that for them ill health is bad health, and there is no way they can notice it unless they clearly remember what it was like to be in good health -making comparisons of before and after- or directly experiencing an improvement that makes them see first-hand the differences between what should be and what you are today. On the other hand, of course, there are also people who are aware that they have a problem and, even if they are not in a position to overcome it on their own at that very moment, recognizing that the problem exists is always the first step in resolving it.

Another reason that hormonal problems are also difficult for many people is that, apart from being seemingly invisible to the sufferer, there can also be confusion about the real problem itself. As hormones influence our behavior and, to some extent, also influence our decision making, we sometimes perform actions that normally, in a normal situation and with a hormonal balance, we would not; this is especially problematic when exposed to the external judgment of other people who are especially toxic. Because you don't behave normally due to hormonal imbalance, people can easily start to believe that it's you and your personality that has a problem; even worse, this issue can also influence your perception and you can get to convince yourself that you have a problem with yourself and your personality, when in reality the root of all the ills with respect to your behavior and your health could be, actually, caused by hormonal imbalance, basically chemical problems with your body. This situation can undoubtedly be detected by several health specialists, including both internist doctors, psychological doctors and nutritionists. One way to know if you're going through this kind of problem is if you're constantly thinking about food, what to eat even though you finished eating a couple seconds ago; think that any situation that has you of low spirits could improve if you eat some kind of sweet -or on the contrary, a good situation deserves something that accompanies him-, you can even get in a very bad mood if you do not have the plate of food you want and, In general, that your life is affected or determined by the choices you make about food, that your life revolves around food.   These are some of the behaviors that are considered extremely toxic to your health and your life, as these can lead to emotional, mental and, obviously, health problems.

A characteristic of people who suffer from pathological anxiety and that this is directed to food and food, is that when they are forced -either by personal decision or external influence- to adopt a new diet or change their diet substantially, it is common for these attempts to end in failed diets and this generates even more frustration. At this point, you have to understand that the problem is not diet like that, but a much more underlying problem: your relationship to food. Arbitrarily forcing yourself to start random diets without any planning and professional consultation represents very high levels of risk to mental and physical health; mental health risks because your planning or approach to diet, among other factors, may not be appropriate to achieve the desired results, which generates frustration and even more anxiety, which only favors and worsens your pathological relationship with food, usually prompting you to make extreme decisions in order to achieve weight loss and generating even more anxiety by wanting to obtain immediate results and ignore - whether consciously or unconsciously- that the slimming process is that, a process, therefore it is progressive and requires a development whose results will appear with the passage of time and persistence in the plan; is also a risk to physical health because the recklessness in pursuing a diet fresh out of the sleeve or you copy a diet that is for someone else, for other purposes, for a specific body, is no guarantee that you will get the same results that are said to be obtained, nor do you know for sure if the plan is even good to start with, this sometimes causes people to diet on the basis of calories only, ignoring the nutritional values of foods, which can be translated, for example, into people dieting on the basis of sweets, sweets and soft drinks, because they are foods that also provide calories and, by the way, are foods to which they are addicted, we can already imagine the negative impacts on health after consuming soft drinks, sweets and sweets for months only.

These problems can become complex and complicated depending on the case of each one. This difficulty is sometimes invisible to many people because they believe that everything can be achieved on the basis of willpower and many desires, ignoring that the will, beyond being something ethereal and abstract that lies within us, is rather the product both of all our experiences that shape our lives, as of all their processes that occur supported by a biological organism whose multitude of interdependent and systemic elements and mechanisms condition and determine the way in which the will, the mentality, the conscience and the behavior are manifested: that is, our will is directly related not only to abstract and biological mental aspects, but to the totality of our organism. Rather than excuse, the above is to understand what are the factors that come into play to sabotage our real interests and to be able to do something about it, understanding also that, as it is a condition sometimes pathological, anxiety can sabotage the desires of the will; for this very reason, it is dangerous to make so many sudden changes in an arbitrary way in our diet.

The consumption of food for anxiety is a fairly common condition and especially in recent years, with a progressively high trend. The best thing if you consider that this condition may be your case is that you go to psychological help to solve problems that go beyond appearances, how your body looks, because there are psychological processes -and even, cultural and social- which must be taken into account when undergoing some kind of treatment. In many cases, eating anxiety is just a manifestation of unresolved internal problems some time back in your life, so there's a chance that eating anxiety is just the tip of the iceberg of a deeper problem.

Recommendations for Eating Anxiety

Although this problem can become complex and complicated, without this being solved with some magic formula, we can give some recommendations to better deal with an unfavorable situation. These tips are designed so that you can stick to them in a simple way and that you can develop a bit of superficial control over your anxiety. The precondition for this to work is to make the decision to do so, even if it is difficult, because we are in a learning process: every improvement process is a learning process, so it is natural that we may fail. In this sense, if we feel insecure to the point that we have an emotional attachment to food, little effective will be our efforts if we do not manage to be honest with ourselves and begin to know and address conflicts

- The first thing we can take as advice is the recognition of the current situation, the identification of the moment you are in the present, stop for a couple of seconds before executing any action that drags us into the vicious circle. In these cases it is essential to adopt the five-second method. What does this method consist of? Wait and count to 5 each time we go to do something about the food, either buy it, order it online, cook it, prepare it, eat it, etc. Whenever we go to do that impulsively, let's stop for a few moments and count to five. That's it. Even if you have the sandwich in your hand just to get into your mouth, if you managed to stop, you're doing fine! The next thing is to ask a series of questions: why are you going to eat what you are going to eat? Do you feel bad about a low blood sugar, or does your body really say you're hungry? Are you sure that the feeling of hunger you feel is truly hunger, or the anxiety you are feeling and is controlling your behavior? Are you feeling bad, frustrated or stressed out and that's why you want to eat?... The purpose of this advice and exercise is to awaken your awareness, it is to make it easier for you to realize what are the moments when these episodes/moments of anxiety hit the door and intake occurs. Identifying these moments is crucial to our progress and improvement, even if in the end you have decided, after applying the five-second method, to eat the dish in the same way. Yes, even if we "fail" to avoid eating at that time, the real purpose is to get to know each other. If by the way you manage to avoid consuming, it is also valid and fine! We strongly advise you to carry some kind of diary or notebook in which you will write down what are the moments and hours of the day in which you go through these moments of anxiety, write down how you felt before, during and after the moment, and try to identify and describe what you think took you or triggered the episode. You can even consider it a kind of diary, and the description of everything that happens, including our feelings and especially feelings, is important to fulfill the purpose of this first advice. ¡ Cheer up!

-

- In the case of food being used as a kind of hobby or as a positive reward/reinforcement to reward you for your efforts, even if it sounds tempting, we recommend looking for a more productive or healthy way to make us feel better about achieving goals.

-

- When you feel like eating, it is good to have some water and lemon or some tea. The taste of both drinks can soothe your craving for food and create some satiety without the disadvantage of having ingested excess sugars or calories.

- Sleep is a natural process that allows us to regulate the chemicals in our bodies, including hormones. Sleep deprivation causes irritability in people, which in some ways also implies greater sensitivity and/or volatility of emotions. You can already imagine what this means for emotions like anxiety and stress and how this will impact your behaviors, especially those related to unhealthy eating habits.

-

- Since we have been talking so much about the importance and role of hormones and chemicals in our bodies, it is time to mention serotonin. This hormone/chemical basically contributes to your feeling of well-being and happiness. Low levels of serotonin will imply a greater difficulty to feel happy and to seek meaning to the things of life; high levels of serotonin, on the contrary, contribute to higher levels of well-being and happiness. The cases of people suffering from bipolarity are mainly due to an imbalance of this chemical, making its instability -sometimes high and sometimes low, sometimes medium-end- generate sudden changes in the mood of people. The natural thing is that this chemical is at normal levels and that certain alterations occur when something produces sadness or happiness without this resulting in a neurological pathology. For this reason, exercise is a natural source of serotonin and even dopamine. For this it is not necessary to jog for three days without stopping just to secrete more serotonin. We recommend starting to adopt short-term exercise routines, as these are able to generate the same effects in our mood, and if you are not a person very dedicated to physical activities, this is a good alternative! The release of serotonin through exercise will help to control the levels of anxiety and stress that your brain is secreting, favoring the chemical and/or hormonal balance of your body and improving your well-being and happiness with yourself in general, helping you better appreciate things around you or yourself. However, if you are a person who has some pathology that directly or indirectly affects the production of serotonin, or simply no type of activity generates some happiness, we recommend, as always, attending professional help. This is also our last piece of advice.

- All the problems we have with our behavior and the way we act and relate to the world can have their origin in some kind of disorder. Knowing if we have any kind of problem means that we can solve it or at least know how to lead our life without our mental conditions being an impediment to carry it out according to our will and our desires. In this case, the ideal scenario is that if you suspect that you suffer from anxiety at pathological levels
- you go directly to

professional help to improve your relationship with food, or with anything else that is negatively affecting you!

Intermittent fasting is a powerful ally if you are a person who wants to improve your lifestyle. The possibilities are quite high that you can better control your anxiety through intermittent fasting and with the necessary professional assistance, backed by the effort and perseverance that will allow you to overcome that first great obstacle. On the other hand, if you are very excited to start and want to go at the speed of light, but at the same time, you feel that your condition affects you too much during the process generating even higher levels of anxiety, It is advisable to ease the step and gradually assume the process until you have adopted it in its entirety. Let us remember that, in previous pages of this text, the adoption of intermittent fasting can be both sudden and progressive; always methodical, always adapting to the needs of each one of us.

Long-term or short-term fasting

Discussions are still on the table on how beneficial intermittent fasting can be or whether, on the contrary, its adoption for long periods of time has negative consequences on people's health. In this regard, there are divided opinions; while some experts maintain that relatively extended periods of fasting are important for detoxification of the body and also promotes and induces digestive rest, making it easier for us not to eat compulsively because we can identify when we are eating on impulse or because we are hungry; in the other spectrum of claims, there are specialists who claim that fasting represents a stress situation for the organism from a metabolic point of view, and that for this reason the hours of fasting should not be exceeded beyond the natural periods of our animal activity -night fasting-. If fasting is extended, this could cause problems related to the psyche, behavior, and emotions.

Undoubtedly there are opposing arguments on the side about the length that should have intermittent fasting in the food of people, because there are people who have experienced first hand for years who affirm the health benefits of this modality. Despite this, the experts have not been able to decide.

Given the uncertainty about the decision of the experts and the benefits that many people have experienced, the most recommended will always be to see how your body reacts once you know how it works and responds under certain situations. You are the person who best knows the limits of your body, be aware of what you need and what you are supposed to do. Depending on how you and your body are, intermittent fasting cycles could last a couple of months or even more years; you can apply it for the rest of your life or only at certain times, in order to detoxify your body if you went to a party and ate too much junk food.

The changes we'll see throughout the fasting process aren't just about weight variation and whether you look slimmer. Since we are talking about one of the main sources of life for us, it means that our whole body will be affected to a greater or lesser extent, in some way or another. In this sense it is also good to see the state of the skin and hair, whether they are opaque or shiny. The color of our eyes, specifically the sclera and the tissue behind the skin of our shiners are also indicators of our health. It is essential to be attentive to the signals that our body gives us as reactions to fasting, to record and document everything we observe over time to be able to control the process. This is a good tactic adaptable to any kind of plan, not just those concerning food and fasting.

On the other hand, it is necessary to remember that on many occasions the benefits of intermittent fasting are not immediate. As we have mentioned repeatedly in this text, since it is a process, the transformations inherent in it appear in a progressive way. It is important not to forget that the body must necessarily go through a process of adaptation, whether slow or a little faster than other people, everything will depend on the conditions of your organism. While results and progress may not be visible during the first few weeks, it's not like you'll last months waiting to see what's happening. What actually happens is that your body is changing day by day at a lot of smaller scales in each of its parts. The sum of the totality of all the changes that your body goes through, after having certain advances in the process, is what we will begin to show as the substantial changes on a superficial level. With regard to appearance, it is important to remember that we, on a personal level, will take longer to see the differences and changes than other people will. That is, other people may be able to tell you about the most noticeable changes in your body and you may be blind to them, not notice them at all. This is perfectly natural because we see ourselves every day, and sometimes more than once each of those days. Being so often in touch with our own image, we get used to it to the point that any slight change we do not notice until they begin to be remarkable enough; the same does not apply to other people. If we assume that people see you a few days a week-let's assume 3 times a week-they are more sensitive to noticing the small changes in your body. This does not mean that you will not be able to notice it, but that it will take you a while longer to notice it because you still have a referential image in your brain about yourself. All your brain needs is to get used to the changes it unconsciously begins to recognize. In a similar way the body acts, it recognizes all the changes and although it takes time to react, it will always be on the move and working. ¡ Don't be discouraged!

In cases where you find yourself in a situation where you want or should give up intermittent fasting, we recommend 200% that it be done gradually. The substantial and radical changes that our body goes through will make it react as if under attack, it will trigger the metabolic alarms and we can react negatively. Although the body sometimes delays in demonstrating results, the truth is that it is always in a state of alert and more when sudden changes occur that attack the normality to which it is accustomed -remember, again, the systemic nature of our organism. For this reason, it is important not to trigger your alarms and avoid all excessive stress as far as possible.

Intermittent fasting and cardio-metabolic health

The various studies and experts involved in them on the benefits of intermittent fasting have always been out of tune with each other, especially when we talk about metabolic health.

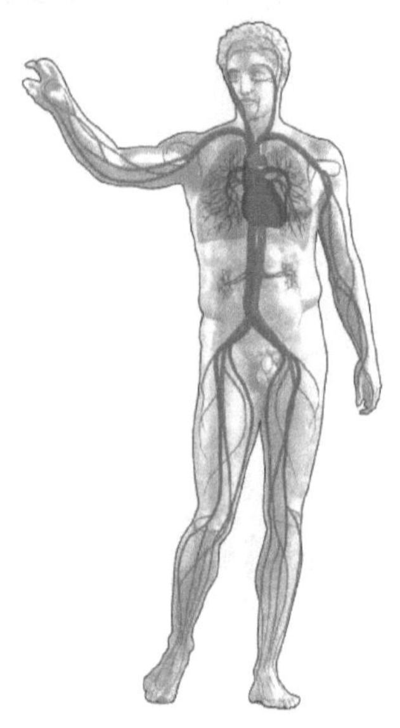

The cardiovascular system is the main carrier of nutrients and resources for our whole body to function properly

To understand the implications of intermittent fasting in relation to metabolic health, you first need to understand what metabolic health is, a matter that many people either through ignorance or resistance are assuming is easy to intuit.

Metabolic health is influenced by various factors. Its status and performance can be measured if five of its variables are within ideal values. These variables/factors are:

- Glycemia/glycemia: This factor indicates the amount of glucose in the blood. Glucose is a fundamental input for the functioning of brain cells and red blood cells throughout our body. Appropriate levels of glycemia refer to the growth and strengthening of our body. On the other hand, the unevenness - whether high or low- of glycemia generate health problems, including diabetic and pre-diabetic problems. In this framework, the blood is able to absorb glucose thanks to insulin, which is responsible for levelling the glucose levels of the body and distributing it as energy to the whole body. Where does insulin come from? Insulin is generated by the pancreas. In the event that we have a bad absorption of glucose, we will begin to raise our triglyceride levels, which is our next variable.

- Triglycerides: the triglyceride variable is responsible for storing fat and these circulate in the blood. They are also known as the adipose tissue that makes up the fat in our body. These have their origin in the fatty acids absorbed from the intestine and come, obviously, from the food we consume and from the liver. The importance of triglycerides is that if they are not at normal levels they can represent a risk to cardiovascular health -in the case that we have low triglyceride levels- or, if not, generate an acute pancreatitis that can endanger the life of the person - in case of having high triglyceride levels-.

- HDL Cholesterol: The Terror of Our Seniors! Cholesterol is nothing more than the fats found throughout our, contribute to the creation of cell membranes and are necessary for the performance of sex hormones. The benefits of cholesterol are equally proportional to its disadvantages if found in excessive levels in our body, causing the main arteries to become saturated with fat in their walls causing thrombosis.

- Blood pressure: refers to the pressure with which blood travels through the artery walls. The blood pressure is measurable starting from two moments of its transit, which corresponds to the two numerical values that represent it. Systolic pressure and diastolic pressure; the first corresponds to the pumping of blood by the heart, while the second refers to the moments when the heart is at rest. High blood pressure is when the systolic pressure has to make a lot of effort to pump the blood because it requires the heart muscle to pump blood even faster within normal operating parameters, representing one of the greatest cardiovascular risks.

Waist circumference: it is commonly believed that the problem of abdominal fat is entirely aesthetic because it takes us out of our proportions and damages our figure. Contrary to this belief, the real problem with abdominal fat is that its accumulation does not only occur in the muscles of the abdomen, but there is also the possibility that the accumulation of fat occurs in the vital organs that inhabit that area, increasing the risk of cardiovascular problems.

Cardio-metabolic risk: the role of intermittent fasting

Clarified the above, we can already begin to point out certain obvious things regarding cardio-healthmetabolic: people with these problems are likely to have type 2 diabetes. The trigger for this disease can be found in conditions such as high blood pressure, obesity and overweight, hyperglycemia, sedentary, smoking, among other disadvantages.

Among the purely cardiovascular benefits that have been reported from intermittent fasting, we have:

- Cell renewal: At this point, cells go from being in a growth mode to a repair mode when they are food-restricted. We have already mentioned this process: autophagy. When cells enter this mode of repair, they go through a more comprehensive self-regulatory process for the removal of their damaged parts. In this process of renewal, the cells begin to generate the capacity to increase their resistance to stress. In other words, they become more resistant to disease.

- The organs begin to release from fat and begin to reduce the volume of fat throughout the body. If you've ever heard of a heart or a fatty liver, this is the part of it.

- It promotes and facilitates the decrease of heart rate when we are in a state of rest. In this sense, it is sometimes considered that intermittent fasting is capable of generating an effect similar to exercise in our heart.

- Lower the Framingham score. This refers to a 10-year projection study on the cardiovascular health of patients. The more points you score in this study, the more likely you are to have cardiovascular disease over 10 years. Some cardiologists have reported a decrease in Framingham's score after having adopted intermittent fasting over six months.

Apart from all the above, there are doctors studying the hypothesis of the metabolic switch This switch consists of using ketonic bodies instead of glucose, bringing two great benefits for the human body: an improvement in cardiovascular protection because some types of ketones have a protective capacity that surrounds the cardiovascular area, improving the chances of survival if the person lasts a long time without eating food, which is equal to improving performance and cardiovascular resistance in general; on the other hand, they also speak of an improvement in metabolic flexibility, referring to the indistinct use of both glucose and ketones without this implying a collapse of the system. The latter benefit appears after at least six months have elapsed since the adoption of intermittent fasting.

Impact on the brain.

Faced with intermittent fasting, the brain has a very particular behavior compared to the other organs: it is the only one that does not shrink in its size. The provisional explanation that some experts have given is that the brain is the one that should best act in stressful situations, such as stress in organisms caused by food deprivation, and this is a behavior that is attributed to our evolution as a species that, Unlike other animals, our development was predominant in this organ. Here are some of the reported effects of intermittent fasting on the brain:

- Improves alertness, motor skills and coordination ability.

- It promotes neurogenesis: the generation of new brain neurons in specific parts and areas of our brain.

- Brain inflammation decreases during the period of food deprivation.

- It increases the stress resistance that the central nervous system may suffer, as protective consequences of some ketonic bodies that help prevent vascular brain accidents.

- It drives neural stimulation and its flexibility.

- It contributes to emotional stability and balance, as we have explained above.

Common errors.

In the process of adopting the new habit it is where we should be most careful to make mistakes because we can adopt them as part of our routine. This makes unlearning the bad habits of intermittent fasting an additional and a little heavier task, because basically we have to make a kind of mental reconnection and replace what we have already been learning. Among the most common errors that we must avoid executing are:

- Do not consume water or not consume enough. One of the reasons people avoid drinking water during periods of fasting is because they mistakenly consider that water goes into things you can't consume. As we have already mentioned about the benefits of drinking water, we will not dwell on this topic. Just remind them that during fasting hours it is more important than ever to keep the body hydrated.

- Insufficient consumption of fiber and vegetables. Both foods are extremely important to protect our digestive system and ensure its proper functioning, in addition to containing nutrients needed for any healthy diet.

- Insufficient consumption of protein. To prevent the body from burning muscle as an energy resource, it is important to keep us stocked with protein at the right times. It is often thought that protein should only be in one meal, whether it is breakfast or lunch. The ideal is to distribute the total daily consumption of protein throughout the three meals, so we also prevent the sudden saturation of them in our body. Other factors that encourage an adequate intake of protein is that they increase satiety levels when eating because it takes your body even longer to digest, while burning extra calories.

- Sleep deprivation. Failure to sleep produces hormones that increase appetite; sleep produces hormones that satiate appetite. Pretty simple, isn't it? Sleep disturbance results in an alteration of this hormonal imbalance, prompting us to eat more food than we should. Little sleep directly implies having greater difficulties of enduring all the hours of fasting. Because you spend more time conscious/awake and burning even more energy resources. On the other hand, it also affects your weight loss because by being in a calorie deficit mode and not sleeping properly, the body will begin to consume muscle mass instead of fat mass.

Optimizing our sleep periods

Sleep plays a fundamental role in all our processes, including slimming or improving our health. Sleep problems are multifactorial. They can be consequences of bad sleeping habits, bad sleep habits, hormonal problems, psychological, among many other elements. If your case is of a pathological condition, such as serious sleep disorders, as is customary, it is best to consult with

the relevant doctor or specialist. We
will then offer general tips to help
healthy people sleep better.

- Create a regular
  schedule. The
  improvement of our
  begins with the creation
  of a sleep habit, starting
  with the hours at which
  we go to sleep and at
  which time we wake up.
  If we force ourselves to
  go to bed at specific
  times, the body, little by
  little, will understand
  these signs as "it's time
  to sleep".

- Avoid emotional excitement. If we get scared, fight, get upset, obviously it will be harder for us to sleep because our body is in a kind of stress. That is, we find ourselves unbalanced, so to speak. Avoid watching movies, discussing, or performing activities that stimulate us enough to sustain alertness.

- Exercising constantly uses more energy in our, making us want to replenish it overnight.

- Bathe with hot water. This favors distension and relaxation of the muscles.

- Avoid coffee at least 4 hours before sleep or at night.

- Do not eat so early, because when we sleep will give us hunger, or so late, because the body will be busy doing digestion.

There are other evils that harm our sleep, especially those that occasions physical pain in the neck and back, consequences of a bad posture or surface in which we sleep. In this regard, we recommend:

- Sleeping in a fetal position makes it easy to rest your back, spine and neck in a correct position.

- If you are of the people who sleep upside down, for ergonomics reasons, we recommend placing a pillow under your knees to accommodate the lumbar position.

- Otherwise, if you sleep upside down, the pillow should be placed at the height of the stomach.

Diet Plan.

What is a meal plan? When it comes to food plans, a list of foods, a few menus and hundreds of restrictions comes to mind: goodbye to everything you once liked. In other words, a food plan is a full-fledged diet by far, but the truth is that it is not necessarily so.

Diets are usually recommended or performed for relatively short periods of time, so it's rare to hear someone on a diet say they've been on the same diet for two years. That's the main difference, the food plans are extremely flexible to every taste and need something that the diet does not have, plus the plans are usually more a change of lifestyle and relationship to food than a simple menu that should be followed. This is why creating a standard meal plan for everyone is a serious mistake, it is impossible for a single plan to serve your whole family or even two people.

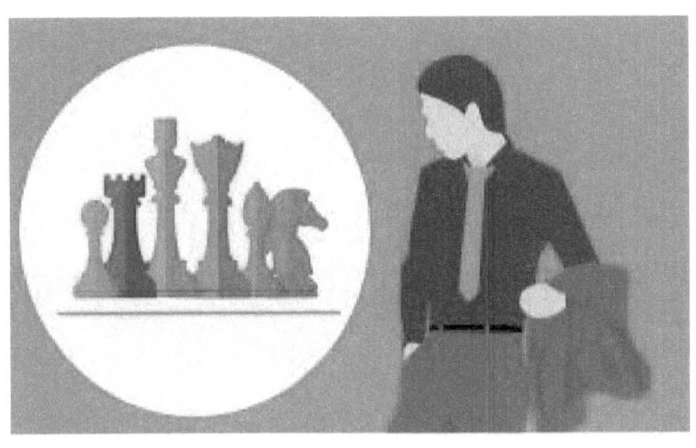

Plans should always have a clear goal to meet. Without a goal, whatever the plan may be

The factors we must take into account when making these food plans are basically everything that has to do with you, your physical condition and your diet:

- Age: A person in his or her twenties definitely does not have the same food needs as an eighty-year-old. This is an important factor that will help to focus the plan on the deficiencies or deficiencies that are according to the age range, for example: an older person should not eat fat while a teenager can ingest them quietly.

- Gender/sex: although many people do not believe it, a female body is not the same as a male body. Each body is different and even more so when we talk about women and men. The body of the woman is formed physiologically to give life, which certain changes or eating habits could generate fatal hormonal changes that on the contrary would not affect the man.

- Health conditions: Of course health conditions can change a lot the food plans of everyone, there are people intolerant to lactose, diabetic people who cannot consume large amounts of food and many other conditions that can make your eating plan completely different from others.

- Physical activity: It is important to keep in mind that people will eat different amounts depending on the physical activity they do. A high-performance athlete will usually consume far more calories than a sedentary person who does not exercise regularly.

- Type of food: Nowadays it is very common to find vegans and vegetarians, clearly people who carry this type of food will not have the same food plans as people who consume products of animal origin. This is a very important factor when planning.

- Food Tastes: Tastes are something that many people don't care about when planning a change in their lifestyle and diet. It is common for people to suddenly give up what they like and condemn themselves to eating chicken breast and broccoli for weeks. This should not be so! It is extremely crucial to know what we like and what we do not and so find a food plan that will satisfy us in every way. The food also exists to give us good feelings and to transmit tranquility, it should not be a fight to eat that last piece of broccoli that we do not want.

Now we are going to talk about two food plans that do not at all encompass a totality of what should have the food of each person, remember that all the factors that we have mentioned above must be applied to each particular case.

People who come to intermittent fasting usually look for a weight loss or want to find a way to stay at their current weight, so let's split the next section in two.

Eating plan to lose weight with intermittent fasting.

When we're looking to lose weight, one of the main things we need to do is get into a calorie deficit. What does this mean? That based on the amount of calories that each person should consume daily, we should either consume less or burn more through exercise. What about intermittent fasting? By itself with this method we are reducing the amount of time in which we eat, which has the general consequence of decreasing a little the amount of calories normally. It is not the same to eat for 16 hours than to eat for 8 hours, the amount of food we can ingest is definitely less.

Assuming that your intermittent fast is night and day, meaning that you don't eat at night while you sleep, and you don't eat during the early hours of the morning, we can say that breakfast doesn't exist in your day, Starting from this we will talk about the most ideal meals you can have during lunch and dinner. Keeping in mind that this plan is for weight loss.

Lunches:

It is important to consume proteins, fats and, if you prefer, carbohydrates. These three macronutrients will help you to keep your body functioning, depending on the type of diet you prefer (ketonic or carbohydrate) the amount of these macronutrients will vary, however, here we will give ideas that encompass everything a little.

- Grilled chicken with green vegetables that grow above the ground, you can season with olive oil, salt and pepper any other low-calorie and if possible, as natural as you can. Let's avoid dressing with too much processing.

- A lean piece of red meat with brown rice and vegetables that grow above the ground.

- Legumes such as lentils, chickpeas, caraotas or some

other grain with lots of vegetables.

- Some cream of vegetables that grow under the ground, these are usually the ones that contain the most calories and carbohydrates so it is advisable to eat them alone or with some food very low in calories.

- Some fish like salmon, tuna or prawns, these are very good, nutritious and in addition to the healthiest there are. These accompanied or alone are ideal for a good lunch, they can even be accompanied by some starch vegetable like potato. In moderation!

Remember that there are many recipes on the web that will help you to see your food much more varied and healthy, not everything is more vegetable protein on the plate. You can manage to make a low-calorie pizza or lasagna.

Avoid excess oils and any sweetened or processed drinks. The ideal thing to lose weight is to consume natural, fresh meals and no sausages and this type of foods that contain many ingredients that are usually harmful to health or have excess calories.

What about the candy?

There are many much healthier options that serve to kill your sweet tooth: coconut flour instead of wheat flour, dark chocolate instead of milk chocolate, splendour instead of sugar and so on. If you want to eat dessert the ideal thing is to make them at home with these healthier ingredients and have a good calculation of the calories of each serving.

Dinners:

During dinners we must avoid the whims that we can give ourselves during the afternoon, that piece of dessert or the starches or legumes that we can afford during the day, at dinner time the ideal thing is to avoid it and concentrate on the most healthy food, low in calories and easy to digest.

Cauliflower rice, there are many recipes on the web, but it is as simple as grating the flowered part of the cauliflower and then boiling it for cooking. The result will be a kind of rice, but low in carbohydrates. You can mix this with pieces of chicken and some vegetables.

Tuna or shrimp salad. You can add the vegetables you like the most looking for always that are starch-free: eggplant, cucumber, zucchini, onion, etc. Avoid the potato and carrot in this salad. You can season it with olive oil and even lemon.

Omelette with eggs or scrambled eggs. Egg is a very complete food that provides a lot of benefits. Eating two or three eggs for dinner in the way you like best is always a good option.

Eating plan to maintain your ideal weight

It's important to know that to maintain weight, unlike to lose weight, you need to consume the exact calories or be in a very small calorie deficit. While maintaining weight for many people is extremely difficult, as they tend to gain weight or lose weight, these small weight variations are completely normal and should not be a major conflict.

The good thing about this eating plan is that it certainly has a lot more possibilities and is more open to change than plans to lose weight. However, it is important to know the limits and not get carried away by the relaxes that involve a maintenance plan.

Moderate portions of pasta and rice can be added for lunches, if they are whole grain even better. You can consume a little more condiments and even occasionally some sauce such as mayonnaise or tomato sauce.

Cheeses are something that should normally be consumed very carefully as they contain many calories, however, for a maintenance plan this consumption can be more extensive and relaxed. The ideal is to consume cheeses without carbohydrates like mozzarella.

Fries are something that should be banned, but they're definitely delicious. If your idea is to maintain yourself you can give yourself these tastes very often and moderately, since, although a day of fried foods will not make you fat, a few days will add a few grams that will vary your weight and also affect your health.

At dinners you can allow starches and some flours from time to time, although ideally avoid them during these hours as the body will take longer to process them and you may feel heavy during bedtime.

In general both plans are quite comprehensive and do not seek at all to serve you as a detailed guide or as a diet to follow, they are simple ideas that you can use to broaden your horizons or to understand a little better how it should be. Remember the factors we mentioned at the beginning and look for the best food plan that suits your needs. Each body is a world and each world has different factors within it that need to be treated with particularity.

Final words.

We have finished reading the text. In this last part of our long journey, you may have noticed that the subject of fasting is much more complicated than stopping eating and then eating again; it goes beyond a simple caloric restriction.

Any change we want to make in our lives will always be difficult to implement at first. When you are new to this eating habit it is normal that it is somewhat difficult to adapt to the new horarioss, especially because we feel that our mind and body are sabotaging our intentions and will. The most important part of the whole process lies in two factors: the first weeks and the constancy after that. The first few weeks are difficult because we are very new to this new dynamic until we begin to get used to it and the level of difficulty has already dropped for us, sometimes we may even find it boring that things have stopped or, on the contrary, relieved that we have reached that point. Thus, in one way or another, we may be tempted to give up fasting because it has already bored us and we believe we have already achieved the purpose, sometimes forgetting that adopting fasting is only a means or an end, being the end then, to improve our well-being and our health. Worse still, we may be tempted to believe that, as we have already established this new habit, it will do no harm if we break the rules only once. But look at this thought, remember that our brain is weak by nature and that's why sometimes you can fall into that pattern: if you've done it once, there's nothing wrong with doing it again, is there? After that, you go back to breaking the new routine.

It is not dangerous to get out of the intermittent fasting routine from time to time, but what is dangerous for your interests is to do it after the first few weeks, when we are still beginning to really get used to eating this way.

It is common for people who start fasting intermittently to come up with some kind of previous problem: low self-esteem, emotional problems, health problems, or even social pressure. These topics are usually not addressed in the texts and sources of information related to exercise and health: usually in these topics we seek to create an atmosphere too positive and distant from the evils that affect us people and that, actually, they do affect our performance. Ignoring these problems often leads to a conscious or unconscious recidivism. This is because they do not put the issues on the table and deliberately decided to ignore them because they "hinder" our process, when in fact it is more important than ever to recognize and know them so that we learn to solve them, to live with them and not to relapse back into the root of our problems. These are problems that should not be buried under a meal or exercise. This deliberate ignorance of these problems is toxic to the world of fitness and health .

The most important thing of all is to accept and recognize that each person is different and has different reactions and processes to carry out. This heterogeneity will no doubt determine how you will carry out your own process of change and what are your strengths, weaknesses, opportunities and threats to this new challenge that you face. It's important to know the story behind your desire for change, your desire for improved health, to ask why you're doing it.

It is important then, not only to know the background of our motivation, but also to know the background of our objective. Is that what you really want to do, makes you happy? What is stopping you?

Before closing it is also essential to understand that human behavior is governed by habits and routines. That's how our brain is designed, and that's how it works. That's why we're so good at recognizing patterns, whether they're real or abstract. Our brain will always seek coherence through repetition, similarity and relationships of the elements. This is as true as with our behavior; always, at different levels, our behavior consists of repetitions, routines, similar things and relationships between some behaviors and others with ourselves, with our problems

If you liked the content of this text, be sure to leave us a comment or a positive review about it. Let us know what you liked the most and what you would like to see more content about. Let's hope text is very useful and enjoyable. ¡ Happy fast!